Naouel Guirat Dhouib
Olfa Hammami
Fathi Ben Abdallah

The Pediatric Residency Curriculum

Naouel Guirat Dhouib
Olfa Hammami
Fathi Ben Abdallah

The Pediatric Residency Curriculum

National Survey Of Pediatric Teachers And Residents

ScienciaScripts

Imprint

Any brand names and product names mentioned in this book are subject to trademark, brand or patent protection and are trademarks or registered trademarks of their respective holders. The use of brand names, product names, common names, trade names, product descriptions etc. even without a particular marking in this work is in no way to be construed to mean that such names may be regarded as unrestricted in respect of trademark and brand protection legislation and could thus be used by anyone.

Cover image: www.ingimage.com

This book is a translation from the original published under ISBN 978-620-6-72201-4.

Publisher:
Sciencia Scripts
is a trademark of
Dodo Books Indian Ocean Ltd. and OmniScriptum S.R.L publishing group

120 High Road, East Finchley, London, N2 9ED, United Kingdom
Str. Armeneasca 28/1, office 1, Chisinau MD-2012, Republic of Moldova, Europe
Printed at: see last page
ISBN: 978-620-8-14333-6

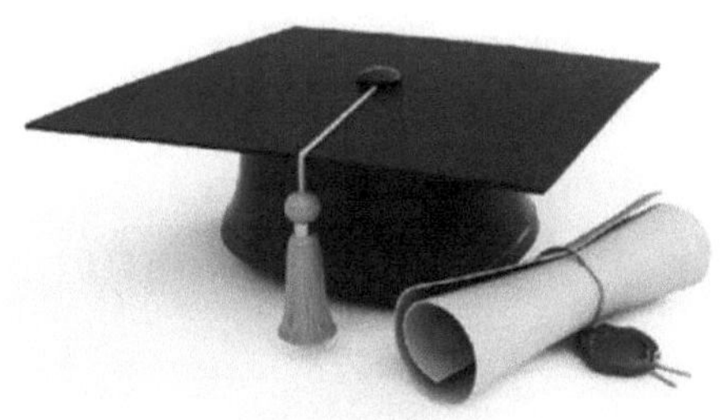

I WOULD LIKE TO THANK ALL THOSE WHO CONTRIBUTED TO THE DEVELOPMENT OF THIS WORK

CONTENTS

INTRODUCTION

Paediatrics covers the whole of medicine for newborn babies, children and adolescents, as well as a number of "sub-specialties". It involves manual processes and the use of instruments. As a result, learning it requires the mastery of several qualities. The development of perfect manual dexterity and the gradual, structured immersion of residents are therefore essential if paediatricians are to be trained to meet the needs of today's healthcare system. The teaching and learning processes must therefore be explicit and predictable in their results.

To improve a curriculum that has been evolving for decades, teachers face a triple challenge [1] :

- Focus training on learning skills rather than simply passing on knowledge, if only because knowledge is multiplying and constantly evolving, and we need to train competent specialists who can act effectively in all circumstances.

- To offer residents learning opportunities that are as relevant as possible to their future working lives.

- Offering all residents the same opportunities to guarantee the principle of quality and safety. fairness.

The aim of this study was to involve paediatric teachers and residents in an experiment to evaluate their theoretical and practical training. In this way, we will seek to bring to light criticisms, both positive and negative, of the current curriculum, and suggest a number of avenues to explore in order to improve certain aspects of this reform of the third cycle of medical studies in paediatrics.

STUDY POPULATION AND METHODS

1. Presentation of the study

This was a cross-sectional and descriptive study, carried out in the form of a survey, among residents and university hospital paediatric teachers. This study was conducted between 23 November and 06 December 2019.

1.1. Inclusion criteria

We included in the study paediatric residents in their 1ère 2ème 3ème and 4ème year, who had completed their medical studies at the 4 Tunisian faculties of medicine, and university hospital paediatricians at the 4 faculties of medicine (Tunis, Sousse, Monastir and Sfax).

1.2. Non inclusion criteria

We did not include in our study residents with less than 6 months' seniority. Before starting the questionnaire, the doctor in charge of the survey explained the purpose of the study and made it clear that the survey would be conducted in a confidential and anonymous manner.

2. Description of the questionnaire (appendix 1)

Data collection waś obtained via a self-administered electronic questionnaire accessible online, created with the Google Forms application in the dedicated site for paediatric residents and sent to teachers by e-mail. Faced with a low response rate, the survey was continued by soliciting participants who did not complete the questionnaire at their places of practice by providing them with the questionnaire in paper format. The estimated time required to complete the questionnaires was 10 minutes.

The items were grouped under six headings with 3 types of question:

- closed questions, most of which require answers to be ticked.

- questions with a judgment

- open questions with free answers.

3. Study statistics

The data were entered using Microsoft Office Excel© and analysed using SPSS© version 19 Windows 7. We expressed qualitative variables as frequencies and quantitative variables as means ± standard deviation, after checking the normality of the distribution, or as median and interquartile range if the normality of the distribution was not checked.The Kolmogorov-Smirnov test was used to verify the normality of the distribution of quantitative variables with a headcount ≥ 50.

RESULTS

1.Evaluation of the paediatric curriculum by residents

1.1.Characteristics of residents who responded to the questionnaire

During the study period, the number of paediatric residents was 168. We received 50 responses after the reminders, giving a response rate of 29.76%.The majority of participants were residents in their 1ère year (32%), followed by those in their 3ème year (30%) (Figure 1). Their average age was 27, with extremes ranging from 26 to 32. There was a clear female predominance, with 36 female residents (72%) versus 14 (28%) male residents, giving a sex ratio of 0.38. The sex ratio for all paediatric residents was 0.4.

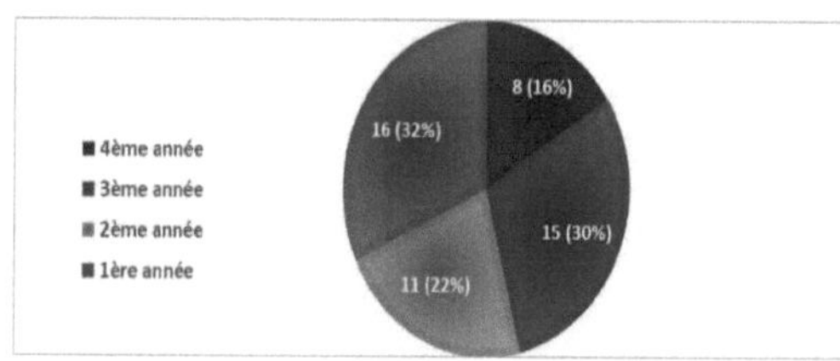

Figure 1: Breakdown of residents by length of service.

1.2.Organisation of training

1.2.1.Perception of the role of residents in training

The majority of residents feel that they play an active role in their own lives. training (Figure 2).

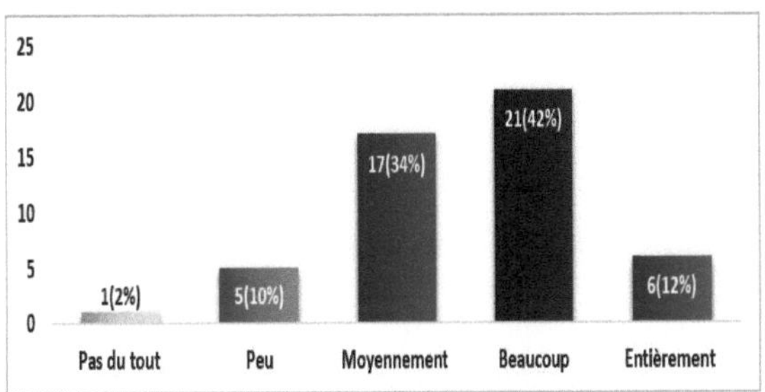

Figure 2: Distribution of residents according to their perception of their own role in their training.

1.2.2. Learning resources

Learning modalities are reported in Figure 3. Nearly 90% of residents reported having received lectures, 68% had participated in clinical case discussion sessions and 66% had participated in other learning modalities, with eight percent reporting mannequin simulation as a training modality.

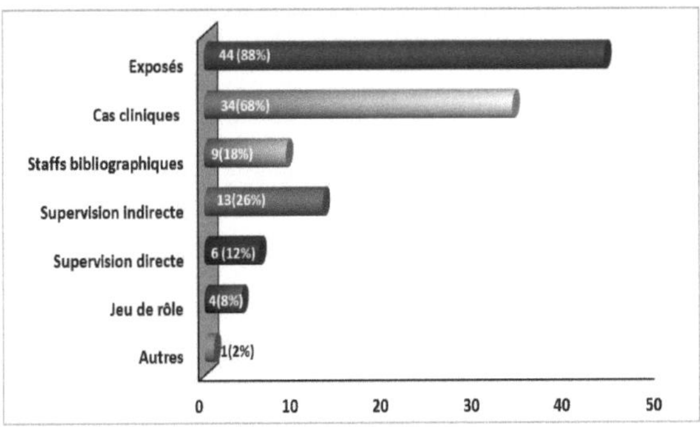

Figure 3: Distribution of residents according to the means used for training.

All the residents had summarised a clinical situation in the form of a clinical observation summary, but only six respondents (12%) had drawn up an account of a complex authentic situation (RSCA).

1.2.3. Perception of the quality of skills development

Most residents felt that the teacher's comments had a positive effect on the progression of their skills throughout their training (Figure 4):

- demonstrating the shortcomings of more than half of residents

- encouraging analysis of their practices

- motivating them to undertake self-training

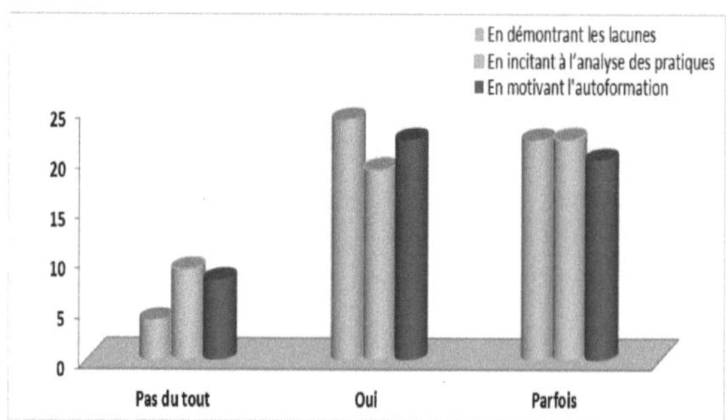

Figure 4: Distribution of residents according to interest in comments by the teacher for their training.

1.3. Assessment methods for apprenticeships

The current evaluation of the paediatric residency curriculum involves a national end-of-specialty examination consisting of an oral and written examination. More than half the residents agreed with this method of assessment (Figure 5).

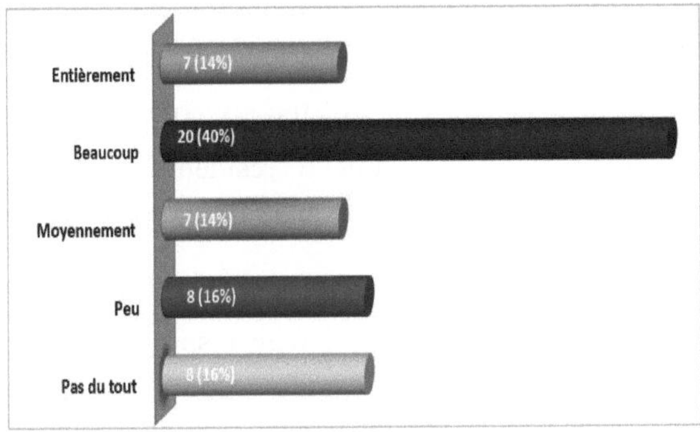

Figure 5: Distribution of residents according to level of agreement with the evaluation now.

Twenty-six per cent of the residents surveyed opted for formative and summative evaluations.

1.4. Type of practice desired by residents at the end of their curriculum

1.4.1. Duration of training

Regarding the desired length of their postgraduate course, the majority of residents: 33 (66%) wanted their residency to last 4 years. Only 17 (34%) residents were in favour of extending the length of the residency from 4 to 5 years. The reasons given by residents are illustrated in Figure 6.

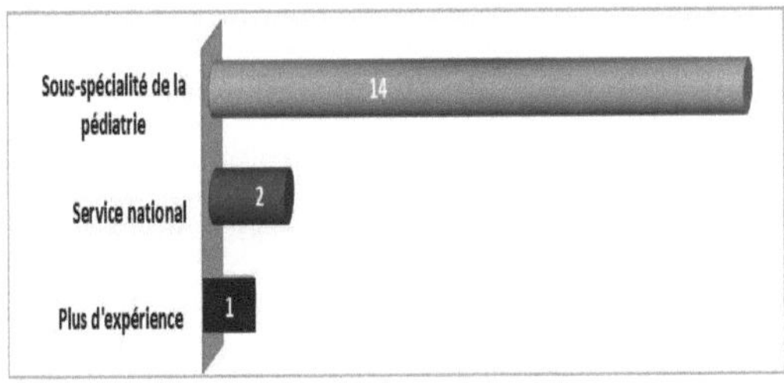

Figure 6: Distribution of residents according to the reasons given for extending the length of their residency.

1.4.2. Number of semesters compulsory

Forty-four residents (88%) felt that one of the six compulsory semesters in the discipline was appropriate, while only 6 residents (12%) would like an additional compulsory semester in their curriculum. The number of residents who considered two semesters in neonatology compulsory was close to those who considered one semester compulsory, with respective percentages of 51% and 49%.

1.4.3. Specialised services

Of the 35 (70%) residents who wanted a specialised paediatric placement in their curriculum, 13 (37.14%) requested a 6-month placement in paediatric intensive care, 10 (28.57%) a placement in child psychiatry, 8 (22.85%) a placement in paediatric neurology, 7 (20%) a placement in paediatric surgery, 4 (11.42%) a placement in genetics, paediatric pneumo-allergology and paediatric emergencies (figure 7). A minority (15 residents, i.e. 30%) who took part in our survey are not agreeing to an internship in a specialist department.

1.4.4. Advanced training course at abroad

Of the residents questioned, 73% considered that doing a placement abroad is an enriching experience in all areas with a great impact on the paediatric training of the resident, while 20% felt that this placement is intended above all for residents wishing to pursue a career in university hospital medicine. In their opinion, this placement would be of little interest to future paediatricians who will be practising general paediatrics. The remaining 7% of residents had decided not to do a placement abroad due to lack of funds and family constraints.

1.4.5. Career guidance

The most attractive career option was a career in a university hospital for twenty-two (44%) of the residents, while 22.4% were considering a career in the private sector and 16.8% had chosen to pursue a career abroad. For the remainder, 11.2% considered the public sector to be their main choice, while 5.6% had not yet made a final decision about their career direction.

1.5.Overall assessment of training

1.5.1. Training theory

The assessment of residents in theoretical training is presented in the figure 8.

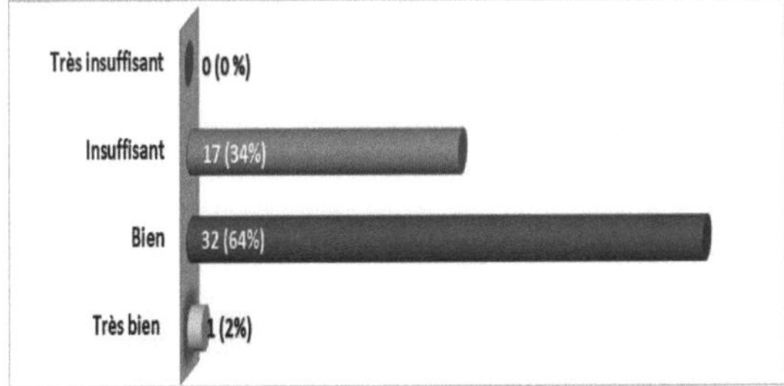

Figure 8: Distribution of residents according to their assessment of theoretical training.

Seventeen percent of paediatric residents felt that they were not satisfied with their progress in theoretical training. They attributed this delay to several reasons summarised in Table I.

Table I: Constraints to progress in theoretical training according to residents.

Reasons for non-advancement	Percentage (%)
Missing courses	53,84
Time constraints	15,38
Lack of support	15,38
No standard protocol for pathologies current	7,7
Lack of motivation	7,7

1.5.2. Training

The majority of residents were satisfied with the quality of practical training. The distribution of residents according to their level of satisfaction with the quality of practical training is shown in Figure 9.

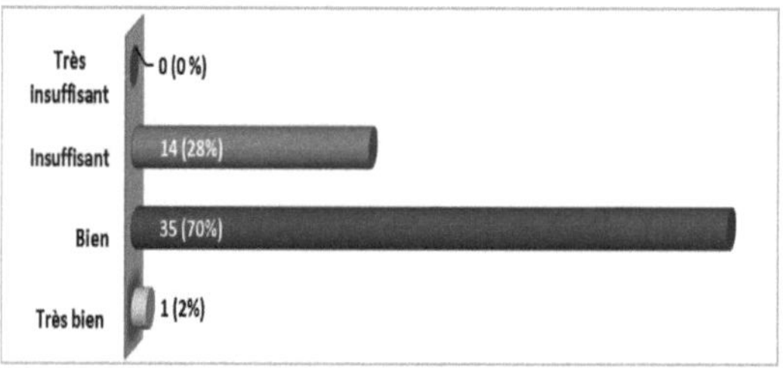

Figure 9: Distribution of residents according to their assessment of practical training.

Twenty-eight per cent were not satisfied with their progress in practical training. They attributed this delay to several reasons summarised in Table II.

Table II: Constraints to progress in practical training according to residents.

Reasons for non-advancement	Percentage (%)
Lack of supervision	33,33
Lack of autonomy	9,52
Time constraints	9,52
Vertical relationship between resident and senior	4,76

1.6. Main difficulties encountered during training

The difficulties encountered by paediatric residents during their time on the wards are shown in Table III. The most frequently cited problems were the lack of critical reflection in training (cited 34 times), the particular difficulties of announcing a serious diagnosis to a child or its parents (cited 20 times) and the education of the child and the family in a context of chronic or rare pathologies (cited 11 times).

Table III: Main difficulties encountered during the course, according to the residents.

Theme	Training type	Deficiencies	Number of quotes
Learning activities	Semiological collection	Data anamnestics	7
	Clinical reasoning for diagnosis Various pathologies	Supervision	5
		Various pathologies	4
	Formulation a Summary of medical observation	Time constraints	7
		Supervision	2
	Prescription from medicines	Guide from medicines	7
Autonomy	Editorial a publication	Autonomy	10
		Guidance	4
		Time constraints	4
	Review of article medical	Reflection criticism in training	34
Communication	Announcement of a diagnosis a serious situation	Training at communication	20
		Fear of reactions aggression	6
	Child education and the family	Difficult for certain pathologies chronic or rare	11

Medical decision	Indication specialised	a	opinion	Relationship vertical senior resident	4	
Practical training	Practical techniques	from	gestures	Time constraints	8	
				Motivation	3	
				Sensation insecurity	2	
				Training simulation	at	1

2.Evaluation of the paediatric curriculum by teachers

2.1.Characteristics of teachers who responded to the questionnaire

During the study period, the number of paediatric teachers was 80. We received 40 responses after reminders, giving a response rate of 50%. Participants were more likely to be assistants (37.5%), but 92.5% of respondents had at least five years' seniority in the faculty (Figures 10 and 11). There was a predominance of women, with 30 women (75%) compared with 10 men (25%), giving a sex ratio of 0.33.

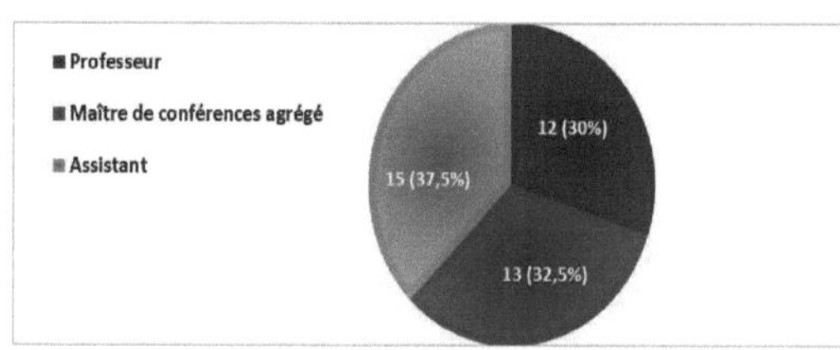

Figure 10: Breakdown of teachers taking part in the study according to grade.

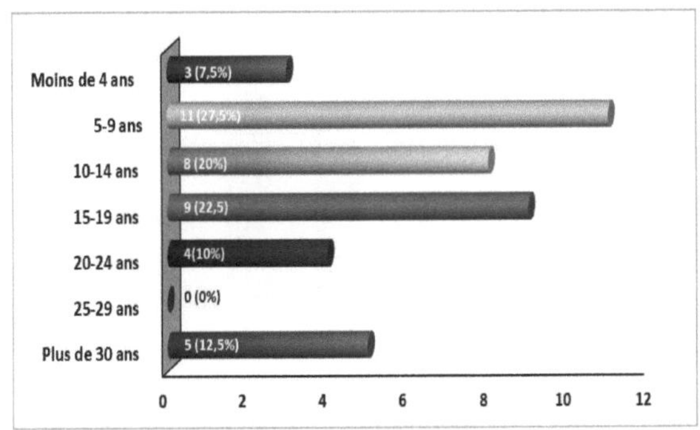

Figure 11: Distribution of teachers participating in the study according to seniority in the faculty.

2.2. Training at internship

2.2.1. Management

Thirty (75%) of the teachers interviewed were supervisors. Of these, only three (10%) were the only people responsible for supervising residents. Supervision was voluntary for 34 (85%) teachers and compulsory for the remaining six. The number of residents per semester and per department as well as the average number of hours per week reserved for supervision is illustrated in Figures 12 and 13 respectively.

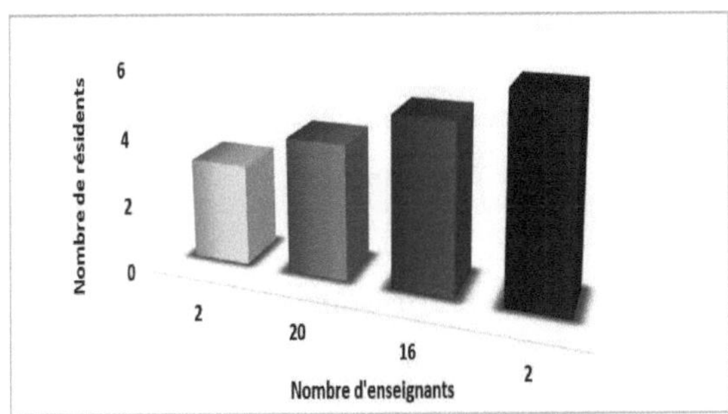

Figure 12: Distribution of teachers according to the number of residents supervised per semester.

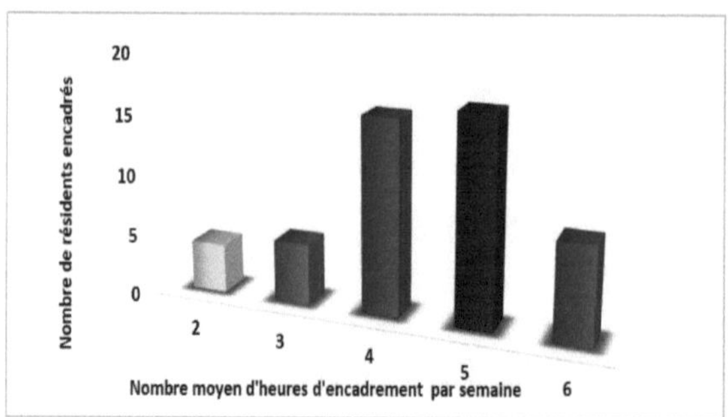

Figure 13: Breakdown of supervised residents by average number of residents hours per week set aside for teaching.

2.2.2. Learning resources (Figure 14)

Thirty-two teachers (80%) used audiovisual means in their training. The majority used a case presentation (57.5%) or a theoretical lecture (47.5%).

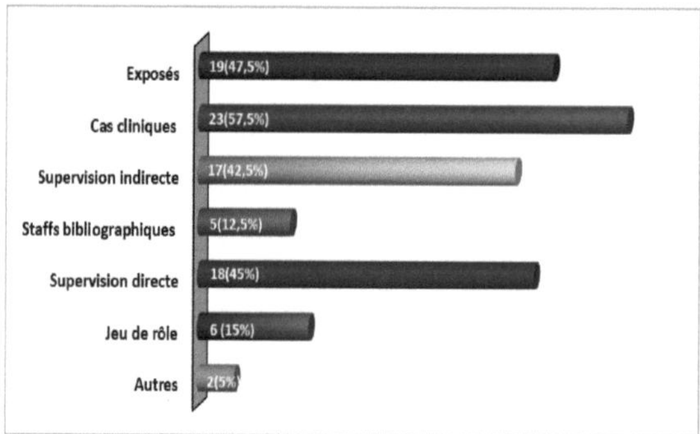

Figure 14: Distribution of teachers according to the resources used for training.

2.3. Assessment methods for apprenticeships

Of the 40 teachers surveyed, 18 (45%) agreed with the assessment arrangements for the paediatric residency programme, which were limited to a certificate examination at the end of the programme (Figure 15). However, 16 teachers

(40%) felt that assessment should no longer be limited to the national end-of-specialty examination. According to the majority of them (13/16), a formative assessment should be scheduled in the middle of the curriculum, in addition to the final certification assessment adopted (Figure 16).

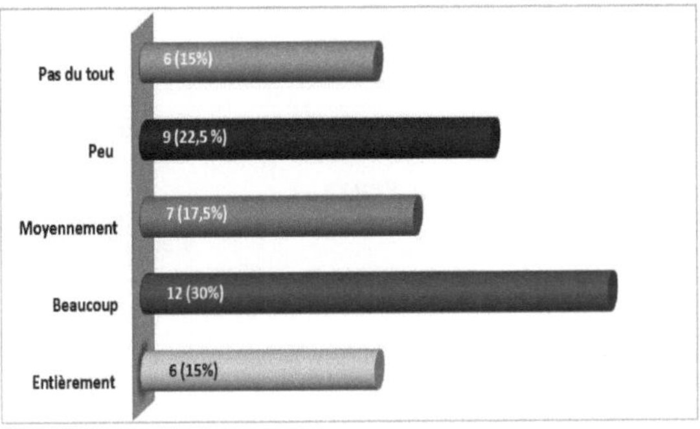

Figure 15: Distribution of teachers by assessment rating current paediatric residency curriculum.

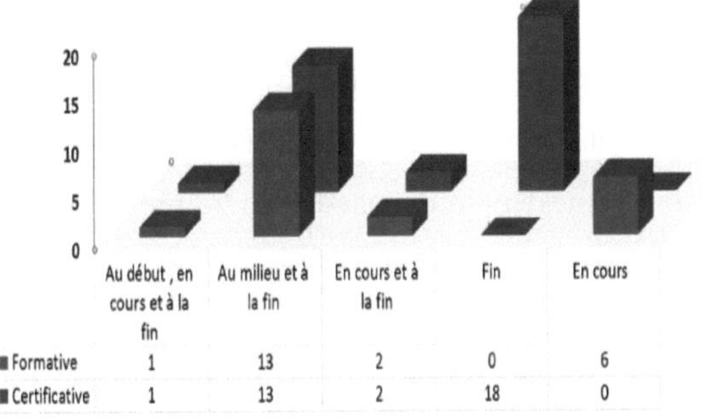

	Au début , en cours et à la fin	Au milieu et à la fin	En cours et à la fin	Fin	En cours
■ Formative	1	13	2	0	6
■ Certificative	1	13	2	18	0

Figure 16: Distribution of teachers by type of assessment.

2.4. Preferences

2.4.1. Duration of training

With regard to the desired duration of the reform of the paediatric residency, 24 (60%) wanted the residency to last 4 years. On the other hand, 16 (40%) were in favour of extending the length of the residency from 4 to 5 years. The reasons given by teachers are illustrated in Tables IV and V respectively.

Table IV: Reasons given for extending the residency period from 4 to 5 years.

	Percentage (%)
General speciality encompassing several sub-specialities	25
Gain more professional experience	20
Paediatrics involves a wide range of pathologies	5

Table V: Reasons given for not extending the residency period from 4 to 5 years.

	Percentage (%)
Sufficient time to manage paediatric pathologies current	35
It's the quality of the work placement that counts, not its duration	5
Service overload	5

2.4.2. Number of semesters compulsory

Twenty-five teachers (62.5%) thought that six compulsory semesters in the discipline was appropriate, while only 6 teachers (15%) would like to see two additional compulsory semesters in the paediatric training curriculum (Fig. 17).

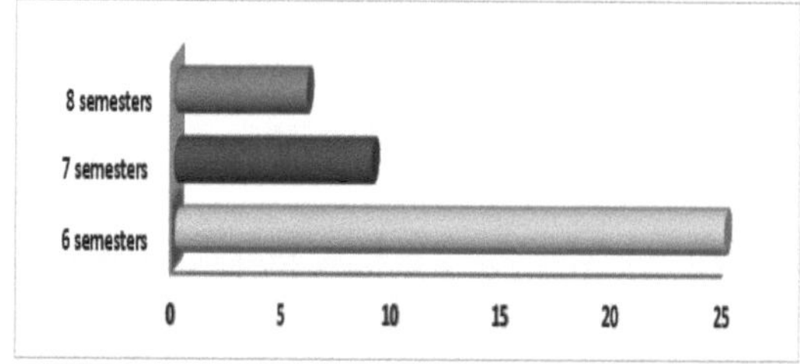

Figure 17: Distribution of teachers according to the number of semesters considered compulsory.

The number of teachers who judged two compulsory semesters in neonatology to be sufficient was higher than those who judged a single compulsory semester to be sufficient, with respective percentages of 57.5% and 42.5%.

2.4.3. Specialised services

Of the 26 (65%) teachers who wanted a specialised placement in paediatrics, 21 (80.7%) proposed a 6-month placement in paediatric intensive care, 16 (61.5%) a placement in child psychiatry, and 10 (38.4%) a placement in paediatric neurology and paediatric haematology. Other services were less frequently proposed by teachers. Some teachers proposed two compulsory semesters in these departments (table VI).

Table VI: Distribution of placements according to teachers' choices.

Specialist department	One semester	Two semesters
Paediatric intensive care	21	1
Paediatric haematology	10	0
Paediatric nephrology	9	0
Paediatric gastroenterology	8	1
Paediatric pneumo-allergology	8	1
Paediatric endocrinology	8	0
Paediatric oncology	3	1
Paediatric neurology	10	1
Paediatric rheumatology	3	0
Paediatric emergencies	8	3
Paediatric cardiology	5	1
Child psychiatry	16	0
Paediatric surgery	8	0
Medical genetics	2	0
Department of Metabolic Diseases	4	0
Adult medicine department	5	0

2.4.4. Advanced training course at abroad

All the teachers agreed on the potential usefulness of a work placement abroad. Among them, 28% considered that a placement abroad was an enriching experience in all areas, with a beneficial impact on the resident's training.

Sixteen per cent felt that this work placement is intended above all for residents interested in a career in a university hospital. The advantages of an advanced training period abroad, as specified by the teachers, are shown in table VII.

Table VII: Benefits of an advanced training course abroad, by type of company teachers.

	Percentage (%)
Enriching training	38
Making paediatrics a sub-specialty	21
Developing professional skills	14
Making the most of your professional experience	12
Acquiring new knowledge	6
Knowledge of other pathologies	2
Mastering a new language	2

2.5. Overall assessment of training

2.5.1. Training theory

Of the teachers surveyed, 85% were satisfied with the theoretical training (Figure 18).

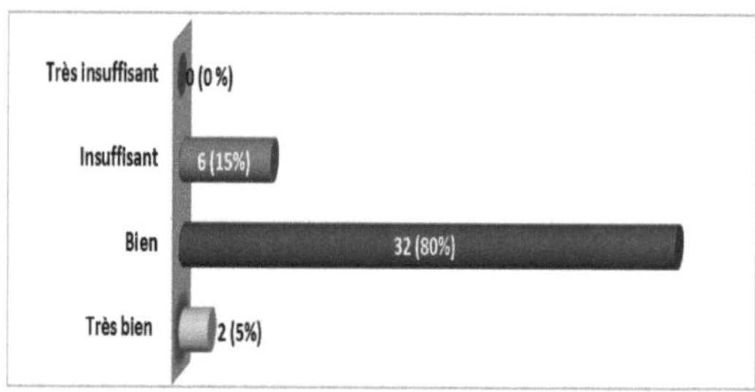

Figure 18: Distribution of teachers by assessment of training theoretical.

The evaluation of theoretical learning activities by teachers is illustrated in Table VIII.

Table VIII: Teachers' assessment of theoretical learning activities.

	Percentage (%)
The methods used favoured the process knowledge appropriation	82
Satisfaction with the quality of the theoretical presentations	75,38
Satisfaction with the quality of clinical cases	70,18
We need to encourage self-learning	25
We need to encourage distance learning	9

2.5.2. Training

Teachers' assessment of practical training is summarised in the figure below. n° 19. Most teachers (92.5%) were satisfied with their practical training.

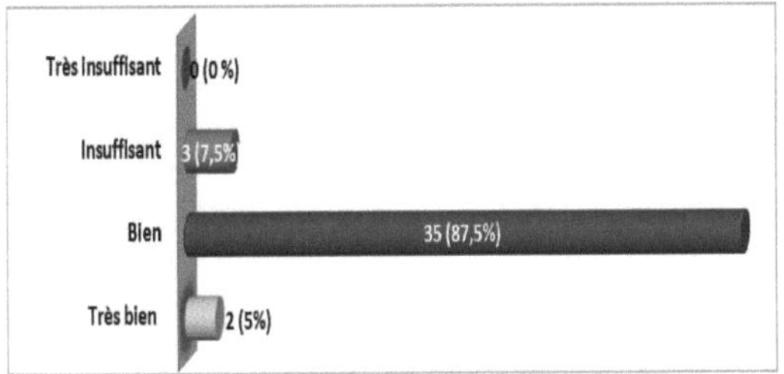

Figure 19: Distribution of teachers according to their assessment of practical training

Teachers' assessments of practical learning activities and their obstacles and limitations are summarised in Table IX.

Table IX: Teachers' assessment of practical learning activities.

	Percentage (%)
Lack of resources for practice	53,84
Satisfaction with the quality of supervision	15,38
Satisfaction with the quality of clinical cases	15,38
Most of the assessment should be practical	7,7
Lack of communication and interpersonal skills	7,7

2.6.Strengths and weaknesses of the course as a supervisor

The strengths and weaknesses of the programme reported by the teachers in response to the open questions are shown in tables X and XI respectively.The strongest points cited were: helping to motivate residents (42.5) and feelings of self-efficacy (20%). The teachers' comments, limitations and suggestions were as follows:

- time constraints

- lack of autonomy on the part of residents

- insufficient logistical resources

- environment unsuited to training

- organisation sometimes difficult (lack of premises, not all residents present, technical problems with audiovisual resources).

Table X: Distribution of teachers according to their assessment of strengths training as a supervisor.

	Number (%)
Motivating residents	17 (42,5)
Sense of self-efficacy	8 (20)
Learning to manage your working time	5 (12,5)
Understanding residents' needs	4 (10)
Development of self-criticism in exchanges ' with peers	2(5)
Professional development	1 (2,5)
Creation of a dyadic resident-teacher relationship	1 (2,5)

Table XI: Distribution of teachers according to their assessment of points Weaknesses in training as a supervisor.

	Percentage (%)
Time constraints	64
Lack of autonomy on the part of residents	16
Insufficient logistical resources	8
Unsuitable environment	4
Organisation of training can be difficult	4

DISCUSSION

In Tunisia, the training curriculum for paediatric residents is based on a combination of theoretical teaching and, above all, a commitment to patient care. However, no formal assessment of knowledge and skills has yet been carried out, and it is unclear whether progress during training meets educational standards and the expectations of residents and teachers. The use of a questionnaire for our study seemed to us to be the most appropriate way of meeting our objectives. It is also the most widely used method worldwide [2,3]. The great advantage of the questionnaire is that it allows data to be collected from a large number of individuals at a relatively low cost. To widen the scope for respondents to express their views, we opted for closed questions with multiple choices, semi-open questions and open questions where the respondent is free to express himself or herself and put forward ideas that we had not thought of. Nevertheless, processing 90 responses to an open question is extremely difficult. The method of distributing the questionnaire on paper at the time of choosing the internship position enabled us to reach a significant number of residents compared to the initial distribution of the questionnaire via the internet only. On the other hand, distributing the questionnaire during the traineeships (which was the last resort) was ill-advised because most of the residents, being busy at the time, did not have the necessary concentration to answer a questionnaire. It is also possible that there was a selection bias, with the participation of residents who felt more invested in the training, and/or the most dissatisfied residents who wanted to make their opinion known. The response rate to the questionnaire was 39.88% of all the participants included in the survey, which represents a low participation rate. However, the fact that we were able to reach participants from the four Tunisian faculties of medicine gave us an overall idea of the subject, which could be used to guide future teaching or research programmes on the subject.

1. Evaluation of the paediatric curriculum by residents

During the study period, the number of paediatric residents was 168. We received 50 responses after the reminders, giving a response rate of 29.76%. Of the respondents, 23 (46%) were third- and fourth-year residents. The sex ratio was 0.38. This fact is explained by the qualitative demographic change, which is the constant feminisation of medicine and paediatrics [4]. This feminisation was noted in an American study of medical students carried out in 2007 and in a Canadian study of paediatric residents [5]. The results of the questionnaire assessing knowledge acquisition show that daily practice is considered very important for the majority of residents. Theoretical teaching is typically based on clinical cases and lectures. Of the residents surveyed, only 8% said they had taken part in a simulation session on a mannequin as a training modality. Yet simulation in paediatrics has been shown to be an effective learning method for acquiring knowledge and skills useful in clinical practice, enabling theoretical knowledge to be consolidated, technical skills to be developed and interaction between members of a healthcare team to be enhanced [6,7]. This teaching tool was necessary for several reasons [8,9]:

- It is an aid to learning how to make ethical decisions

- It focuses on areas of know-how and interpersonal skills

- It increases the learner's performance from "novice" to "expert".

beginner" then "proficient" level

- It enhances the memory of theoretical data.

- It has a positive impact on patient safety.

Since January 2009, simulation has been considered a compulsory training method for emergency procedures in North America [10]. In France, simulation is now recognised as an official teaching method in medical studies, and is included in the new 3ème cycle of medical studies. medicine and it is planned that paediatric residents will receive simulation training throughout their studies [11]. In our study, the majority of residents agreed with the current evaluation limited to the national examination at the end of the specialty and comprising an oral and written test. However, 26% of residents opted for formative and summative assessments. In France, there is little evaluation of residents' knowledge: 84% do not have any, whereas 85% said they would like to see it introduced as part of their curriculum [12].During the national evaluation carried out by the inter syndicat national des résidents de France, 58% of residents stated that they had not been assessed on their theoretical knowledge of the curriculum [12]. This knowledge assessment could take the form of an annual examination on basic knowledge of general paediatrics and neonatology. Formative assessment promotes both the process of transmission by the teacher and the process of acquisition of teaching content by the student. It enables residents to make progress in their learning and to obtain frequent feedback. The resident will thus be made aware of his strengths and weaknesses, as well as his progress. As a result, the teacher will be better able to respond to the needs identified by adapting his or her teaching methods.According to the results of this survey, the current duration of four years is sufficient to become an expert paediatrician according to the residents questioned. Recently in France, the length of training for trainees in general paediatrics leading to a specialist diploma in paediatrics has been extended to 5 years in view of the diversity of the specialty. In Tunisia, the paediatric residency curriculum takes place over 4 years (8 semesters) following the reform of the third cycle with a minimum of 5 compulsory semesters in paediatrics, 2 compulsory semesters in neonatology and one optional semester among the following specialties: paediatric surgery or genetics or medical imaging or paediatrics or neuro-paediatrics or child psychiatry. In our study, 82.84% of respondents were convinced of the usefulness of an elective, which for the majority of residents would be child psychiatry. This choice can be explained by the increase in psychiatric emergencies in children who are not treated by paediatric emergency departments. In fact, to this day, hospitalisation in paediatrics is determined by somatic indications [13].In line with other studies, the most common career choice was a university hospital course (44%) [12,14]. According to a recent French study of 1215 paediatric residents, 39% planned to work in a hospital, 33% in a combination of private practice and hospital work, 14% in a university hospital, 5% in private practice, 1% in community paediatrics, 1% in other activities (humanitarian medicine, abroad) and 8% in other fields (e.g. paediatrics).% did not yet know. According to the same study, the theoretical teaching of paediatricsseemed insufficiently adapted for 24% of residents, partially adapted for 48 The most common reasons given for this were lack of training in general paediatrics, time constraints and lack of support. The main points made in the comments were the lack of training in general paediatrics, time constraints and the lack of support. Others mentioned the need to use distance learning methods such as e-learning or videoconferencing, and the desire for more practical teaching using high-fidelity mannequins [12]. In our series, theoretical teaching in paediatrics seemed insufficiently adapted for 34% of residents and well adapted for 64%. More than half of the residents (53.84%) were not in favour of online courses. In Tunisia, although access to the Internet is improving, the infrastructure is still insufficient to allow widespread use of e-Learning. This access is characterised by major variations between regions. Other reasons given for residents' failure to progress included the lack of companionship (15.38%) and the lack of national harmonisation of protocols, combined with a lack of motivation (7.7%).In France, the five topics considered most important and for which theoretical training was considered most inadequate by paediatric residents were: child development; physiology of infants, children and adolescents; training in doctor-patient communication; medical law; and setting up in town with practice management [12]. Ninety-three per cent of paediatric residents thought it would be useful to have progressive teaching as they progressed through their residency. Ninety-four per cent of paediatric residents would have liked more teaching on high-fidelity mannequins [12].With regard to training in scientific research, 39% of respondents rated it as moderately important and insufficiently developed during the course of their studies, and 32% as very important and insufficiently developed. A study analysing the level of publication of theses by paediatric residents in France showed that 27.9% of these theses were published in a journal referenced in Medline [15].The Société Française de Pédiatrie recently declared that research training for young paediatricians was one of its priorities [16]. Research makes it possible to revitalise medical specialities and contribute to a better understanding of medicine [12].For the majority of participants in our study, practical training is of great importance. It was judged to be adequate by 72% and insufficient by 28% of participants. of residents. The reasons for residents' dissatisfaction with their training were mainly lack of supervision (33.33%), lack of autonomy and time constraints (9.52%) and the vertical resident-senior relationship (4.76%). Hospital internships provide an opportunity to be confronted with real, authentic clinical situations, enabling an introduction to problem-solving, a fundamental element in the development of professional skills [17].However, learning during internships depends on hospital activity, which can fluctuate from day to day. Excessive hospital duties are a limiting factor, as is the lack of planning for learning, particularly the absence of explicit predefined objectives [18]. The main difficulties encountered by paediatric residents during their time on the wards were the lack of critical reflection in training (cited 34 times), the particular difficulties of announcing a serious diagnosis to a child or its parents (cited 20 times) and the education of the child and family in a context of chronic or rare pathologies (cited 11 times). Jamjoom et al prioritised the difficulties experienced by the residents and classified them as follows: heaviness of the task, amount of knowledge to be acquired, role ambiguity, performance anxiety, competition with peers, feeling overwhelmed by the task, lack of sleep, limited time for personal life and leisure, and lack of support [19-21]. On the other hand, other difficulties are less frequently cited in the literature: stress linked to being supervised and evaluated, confrontation with one's limits, adaptation to frequent changes of context, few electives and guilt about doing something other than medicine [22].

2. Evaluation of the paediatric curriculum by teachers

During the study period, the number of paediatric teachers was 80. We received 40 responses after reminders, giving a response rate of 50%. The majority of participants were teaching assistants, and more than two-thirds of respondents (70%) were teaching assistants and associate lecturers. 92.5% of respondents had at least five years' seniority in their grade. Thirty (75%) of the teachers interviewed were supervisors, of whom only three (10%) were the only people responsible for supervising residents. The majority of teachers (34 (85%)) chose to supervise their residents, while six others were required to do so. According to the results of this survey, the majority of supervisors were assistants. This could be linked to a simple recruitment bias, with a greater number of assistant posts being allocated to paediatrics.Thirty-two teachers (80%) used audiovisual means in their training. The majority used a case-based presentation (57.5%) or a theoretical presentation (47.5%). By definition, an audiovisual medium is a basis, a support or a back-up for auditory and visual methods, which makes it an ideal ally in teaching [23]. These media are multiplying, evolving and modernising. More than half the teachers preferred case-based learning, which reflects their orientation towards active teaching methods. The advantages of using video to teach paediatric dentistry, for example, are: attractiveness, discovery of clinical reality, modernisation of learning, modular learning, accessibility and contextualisation of knowledge [24]. However, the production of multimedia teaching aids can have a number of disadvantages: the complexity of production; professional equipment is needed to produce good quality videos (a camera, a microphone, a stand, editing software, etc.); the cost of production; time-consuming; difficult access for some students who may not have access to the Internet or who do not have a medium on which to play the videos (laptops for example) and the passivity of the audience if the videos are not interactive [25]. Regarding the assessment of the paediatric curriculum by teachers, 16 teachers (40%) felt that assessment should no longer be limited to the national end-of-specialty examination. In their opinion, formative assessment in the middle of the curriculum would have a positive impact on the quality of training. They propose that the examination should be conducted by the Tunisian Paediatric Society, on the same model as the American Board of Pediatrics in the United States and Canada: a 3-hour computer-based examination, comprising approximately 150 multiple-choice questions [26]. The strength of this assessment is that it is both certifying and formative:

- Certificative, because the test reflects the resident's knowledge, and they can compare their results with those of their peers anonymously.

- Formative, because the assessment highlights the weaknesses that residents need to work on to improve their score the following year. Finally, it enables them to assess their progress during their residency.

With regard to the desired duration of the reform of the paediatric residency, 24 teachers (60%) wanted the residency to last 4 years. On the other hand, 16 (40%) were in favour of extending the length of the residency from 4 to 5 years. In Europe, paediatric specialty training is not uniform, with residency periods ranging from 4 to 8 years [27]. Some countries, notably the United Kingdom, have developed a detailed professional reference framework setting out the knowledge and skills to be acquired during paediatric residency training [28]. In France, training in general paediatrics currently lasts 5 years. This training leads to a specialist diploma in paediatrics. Additional training of 1 to 3 years is optional, depending on the sub-specialty chosen [29]. The speciality of paediatrics has become increasingly complex and diverse, and the many subspecialisations require specific skills. At the same time as the specialty is evolving, the medical profession has had to adapt to meet the growing demands for results and quality made by patients and public authorities. The extension of the Specialised Paediatrics Diploma to 5 years will make it possible to better meet current training requirements, to develop a certain number of paediatric specialities by means of an option or cross-disciplinary specialised training, and to formalise on a permanent basis the possibility of completing an outpatient placement [30].

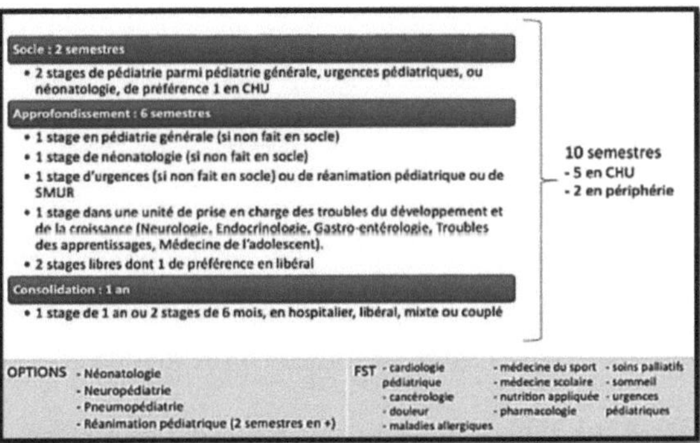

Figure 20: General organisation of the specialist paediatric diploma in France [29].

Of the 26 (65%) teachers who wanted a specialised paediatric placement as part of their curriculum, 21 (80.7%) proposed a 6-month placement in paediatric intensive care. According to the Collège national français des pédiatres universitaires, the content of the paediatric residency is organised into 8 placements, each lasting one semester, 3 of which are compulsory (general paediatrics, neonatology and intensive care or emergency) and 2 of which must be carried out in non-university settings [31].

At present in Tunisia, work placements abroad are optional, depending on the desire and motivation of the resident. The majority of the teachers interviewed were convinced of the potential usefulness of a training period abroad. Among the teachers 28% of those surveyed considered that a placement abroad is an enriching experience in all areas, with a major impact on the paediatric training of the resident. The introduction of a placement abroad in reference centres as an integral part of the curriculum through partnerships with other world-renowned residency programmes may also be a good short-term solution. This experience would enable residents to benefit from other training methods and open up to other perspectives, as well as appreciating the advantages of Tunisian training. This initial survey of paediatric teachers' assessment of theoretical training showed that the majority of teachers were satisfied with their theoretical training. However, 15% considered it insufficient. In our opinion, theoretical training can be delivered via a distance learning platform. E-learning is a training model based on the principle of interaction between tutors and peers and therefore makes it possible to apply the socioconstructivist theories in educational psychology based on the principle of tutoring. The interactions between tutor and learner are the determining factor in the quality and effectiveness of learning, which helps to keep learners motivated. E-learning can be particularly useful for residents of establishments at a distance from training centres or doing electives in other specialities. As far as the means of communication in e-learning are concerned, the communication forum is considered to be one of the best tools for collaborative work at a distance [32, 33].Traditional classroom teaching will be all the more effective if it involves active learning. As most residents are anxious about being questioned individually during a lesson, an interesting idea is to question them collectively using answer boxes. If there is no answer box and there is a wifi network, residents can answer on the internet from their smartphones. Reassessing them at the end of the course enables the teacher to ensure that his messages have been transmitted and gives the resident a first opportunity to test himself, with all the advantages presented in the first part of the repeated assessment. The

Société Française de Médecine d'Urgence (French Society of Emergency Medicine) already carries out training videos. In paediatrics, the video validated by the Société Française de Pédiatrie on the management of cardiac arrest in children has been viewed more than 250,000 times since it went online in 2013, with proven effectiveness in improving the skills of hospital students [34]. The Tunisian Paediatric Society should promote the production of educational videos.For the majority of participants in our study, practical training is of great importance. It was adequate for 87.5% and inadequate for 7.5 of teachers. More than half (53.84%) of the teachers were convinced that there was a lack of resources for practice, while 7.7% thought there were insufficient interpersonal and communication skills. Post-training feedback provided constructive suggestions and highlighted strengths and areas for improvement. It was certainly a spark that opened the door to reflective thinking for the teachers.Through open-ended questions, we gathered the various comments and suggestions made by the teachers. The comments ranged from praise to constructive criticism. It was difficult to analyse the 40 comments and suggestions made by the teachers, all of whom answered this question. The strong points of this training which were most frequently mentioned were: encouraging the motivation of residents (42.5%), the feeling of self-efficacy (20%), learning to manage working time (12.5%) and knowing the needs of residents (10%). Among the weak points in training that need to be improved: time constraints (64%), lack of autonomy on the part of residents (16%), inadequate logistical resources (8%), unsuitable environment and organisational difficulties (4%). Off-campus training is a cost-effective solution that saves time and helps to broaden and improve the quality of education systems.

Finally, our study has a number of limitations:

• a selection bias, since the participation rate was only 29.76%; a better response rate would have reduced this bias and produced more representative results.

• we used only one evaluation tool (the questionnaire). The advantage of this method is that it is simple, easy to use and anonymous. Its limitations are that it is a closed, non-interactive technique. At a later stage, the use of other evaluation tools such as focus groups should enable us to better identify and evaluate other factors expressed and felt.

CONCLUSION

In this work, we identified the needs and assessment of theoretical and practical training in paediatrics based on the views of teachers and paediatric residents. This was a cross-sectional study carried out by means of a questionnaire survey. The questionnaire covered the following topics

- organisation of training

- learning activities

- how learning is assessed

- overall assessment of the course

During the study period, we received 50 responses from residents and 40 from teachers, giving a participation rate of 29.76% and 50% respectively. Women predominated, with a sex ratio of 0.38 for residents and 0.33 for teachers. Thirty-two teachers (80%) used audiovisual means in their training. Nearly 90% of residents said they had received lectures, 68% had taken part in clinical case discussion sessions and 66% had taken part in other learning modalities, including eight per cent who reported mannequin simulation as a training modality.The majority of participants agreed with the current end-of-specialty assessment method. However, 26% of the residents questioned opted for formative and summative assessments, and 40% of the teachers proposed a mid-course and end-of-course assessment.

The results of the questionnaire assessing knowledge acquisition show that daily practice is considered very important for the majority of residents. Theoretical teaching is typically based on clinical cases and lectures.

Theoretical teaching in paediatrics appeared to be insufficiently adapted for 34% of residents and well adapted for 64%. Only 8% of residents said that they had taken part in a simulation session on a mannequin as part of their training.For the majority of participants in our study, practical training is very important. It was considered appropriate for 72% of residents and 88% of insufficient for 28% of residents and 7.5% of teachers. The reasons for residents' dissatisfaction with their training were mainly lack of supervision (33.33%), lack of autonomy and time pressure (9.52%). More than half the teachers were convinced that there was a lack of resources for practice. From the analysis of our results, a number of interesting avenues for action have emerged in order to improve certain aspects of this reform of the third cycle of medical studies in paediatrics. Thus, it would seem worthwhile to :

• use active teaching strategies to improve resident motivation. Active pedagogy places the learner at the centre of the learning system, giving them a number of responsibilities that empower them and improve their motivation and active involvement in their learning;

• encourage the use of new digital technologies for teaching. The use of digital technology makes learners more autonomous, responsive and interested, which is an additional source of motivation.

• Safeguard the necessary theoretical training time ;

• organise teaching on the basis of a professional reference framework, including the theoretical knowledge required to practise paediatrics, but also the knowledge required to practise medicine in its entirety (ethics, medical law, etc.). Our study would reflect the needs of learners and teachers and could therefore represent one of the resources needed to develop this reference system;

• integrate innovative teaching techniques with sustained clinical activity in the field;

• set up a formative and certifying assessment of learning;

• promote the teaching activities of doctors who teach.

REFERENCES

1. Roegiers XE. Pédagogie de l'intégration. Brussels: De Boeck Université, 2000.

2. Gangloff-Ziegler C, Ben Abid-Zarrouk S. Evaluation des enseignements et des formations par les étudiants et construction d'un questionnaire de satisfaction. Actes du congrès de l'Actualité de la recherche en éducation et en formation (AREF), Université de Genève, septembre 2010.

3. Detroz, P. Evaluation de la qualité des enseignements: de la contrainte administrative à l'amélioration des pratiques, Freiburg. 2007: Centre de Didactique Universitaire, University of Fribourg.

4. Women Chairs of the Association of Medical School Pediatric Department Chairs. Women in pediatrics: Recommendations for the future. Pediatrics 2007;119:1000-5.

5. St-Laurent Gangon T, Dural RC, Lippe J, Côté- Bioleau T. Women in paediatrics: The experience in Quebec. CMAJ 1993; 148(5): 773-8.

6. Bullock A, Webb K. Technology in postgraduate medical education: a dynamic influence on learning? Postgrad Med J 2015;91:646-50.

7. Cheng A, Lang TR, Starr SR, Pusic M, Cook DA. Technology-enhanced simulation and pediatric education: a meta-analysis. Pediatrics 2014;133 (5):e1313-23. doi: 10.1542/peds.2013-2139.

8. Oriot D, Boureau-Voultoury A., Ghazali A, Brèque C, Scépi M. Interest of simulation in paediatrics. Arch Pediatr 2013; 20(6): 667-72.

9. Dreyfus SE. The five-stage model of adult skill acquisition. Bull Sci Technol Soc 2004; 24 (3), 177-81.

10. Forbes J. HR 855-A bill to amend the Public Health Service Act to authorize medical simulation enhancement programs and for other purposes. Available on the Internet: URL: https:// www.gpo.gov/fdsys/pkg/BILLS-111hr855ih/pdf/BILLS-111hr 855ih.pdf.

11. Guillois B, Bellot A. Simulation-based health teaching in paediatrics . Perfectionnement en Pédiatrie 2020 ;3 (2):196-204.

12. Girard B, Bendavid M, Faivre JC, Salleron J, Debillon T, Claris O, Chabrol B, Scweitzer C, Gajdos V Theoretical teaching of the Diplôme d'études spécialisées de pédiatrie in France: national evaluation by interns. Arch Pediatr 2017 ; 24 :728-36.

13. Charfi F, Harbaoui A, Skhiri A, Abbès Z, et al. Epidemiological and clinical profile of suicide attempts among children and adolescents in post-revolution Tunisia. Pan Afr Med J. 2019; 32: 204.

14. Mahmoudi A, Noomen F, Nasr M, Zouari K, Hamdi A. Evaluation of the training of general and digestive surgery residents in Tunisia. Pan Afr Med J 2015; 21: 328.

15. Fabre A. Publication of paediatric practice theses. Arch Pediatr 2015;22:802-6.

16. Claris O, Chabrol B. Research work during the paediatric internship: learning to
publish early. Arch Pediatr 2015;22:799- 801.

17. Langevin S, Hivon R. En quoi l'externat ne s'acquitte-t-il pas adéquatement de son mandat pédagogique? A qualitative study based on a systematic review of the literature. Pédagogie médicale 2007; 1: 7-23.

18. Bungener M, Demagny L, Holtedahl KA, Letourmy A. La prise en charge du cancer : quel partage des rôles entre médecine générale et médecine spécialisée ? Pratiques et Organisation des Soins 2009; 3 (40); 191-6.

19. Jamjoom RS, Park YS. Assessment of pediatric residents burnout in a tertiary academic centre. Saudi Med J2018; 39(3):296-300. https://doi.org/10.15537/smj.2018.3.22328

20. Dyrbye LN, Thomas MR, Huschka MM, et al. A multicenter study of burnout, depression, and quality of life in minority and nonminority US medical students. Mayo Clin Proc. 2006;81:1435-42.

21. Gribben JL, Kase SM, Waldman ED, Weintraub AS. A Cross-Sectional Analysis of Compassion Fatigue, Burnout, and Compassion Satisfaction in Pediatric Critical Care Physicians in the United States.Pediatr Crit Care Med 2019 ;20 (3):213-22.

22. Boulé R, Girard G. Residency in family medicine: problems and solutions. Can Fam Physician 2003; 49:472-82.

23. Chávez V, Turalba R-AN, Malik S. Teaching public health through a pedagogy of collegiality, Am J Pub Health 2006; 96: 1175-80.

24. Available at: http://www.creerunoutil.be/- Fiche-11-Avantages-et-

25. Martin W. Creating audiovisual media in paediatric dentistry - 2018 - hal.archives- ouvertes.fr

26. General pediatrics in-training examination. Am Board Pediatr. https://www.abp.org/

27. Pettoello-Mantovani M, Ehrich J, Romondia A, et al. Diversity and differences of postgraduate training in general and subspecialty pediatrics in the European Union. J Pediatr 2014;165(2):424-6.

28. Royal College of Paediatrics and Child Health. Curriculum for paediatric training general paediatrics. https://www.gmc-uk.org/-/media/documents/april-2015-general- paediatrics-curriculum_pdf-60877537.

29. Order of 13 February 2020 amending the order of 21 April 2017 on the knowledge, skills and training models for specialised study diplomas and setting the list of these diplomas and the options and cross-disciplinary specialised training courses in the third cycle of medical studies.   JORF no. 0066 of 17 March 2020. https://www.legifrance.gouv.fr/jorf/id/JORFTEXT000041728662.

30. Chabrol B. Why the city paediatrician will not disappear. Réal Ped 2018 ;221 :41-2.

31. Bacquet M, Bendavid M, Foucambert H, Girard B et al: Reform of the diploma model

d'études spécialisées de pédiatrie : vision des juniors. Arch Pediatr 2016; 23: 784-6.

32. Hollander JE, Carr BG. Virtually perfect? Telemedicine for Covid-19. N Engl J Med. 2020;382:1679-81.

33. Ting DSW, Carin L, Dzau V, Wong TY. Digital technology and COVID-19. Nat Med. 2020;26:459-61.

34. Drummond D, Arnaud C, Thouvenin G, et al. An innovative pedagogic course combining video and simulation to teach medical students about pediatric cardiopulmonary arrest: a prospective controlled study. Eur J Pediatr 2016;175: 767-74

Evaluation of the paediatric curriculum by residents

1/ Seniority in residency grade

- 1ère year

- 2ème year

- 3ème year

-4^{èm}e year

2/ Please indicate your age ? 3/ Gender

Male

Female

4/ Do you feel you have an active role in your paediatric training?

	Not at all	Little	Medium	Many	Entirely
Level of agreement					

5/ What learning methods did you experiment with during your residency?

LECTURES (theoretical presentation by a teacher) CASE STUDY (discussion of a clinical case) Bibliographical Staffs

Direct supervision (constant presenceof the teacher who supervises the residents,giving them direct instructions and checking that tasks are carried out).

Indirect supervision (without the constant presence of the teacher-supervisor)

Role-playing (staging a problem situation involving characters with a given role, under the supervision of a facilitator)

Other (please specify)

6/ Have you written authentic accounts of complex situations?

Yes

No

7/ Do you receive feedback from your mentor on your reflections?

Systematically

Sometimes

Never

8/ Do you feel that the comments of your mentor help you to progress in your training?

	Not at all	Yes	Sometimes
By showing you what you lack			
By encouraging you to analyse your practices			
By motivating you to undertake self-training			

9/ What is your opinion of the current assessment system: a single exam at the end of the course?

	Not at all	Little	Medium	Many	Entirely
Level of agreement					

If you are not satisfied, give suggestions for improvement

10/ What difficulties do you encounter at the end of your course (for 4ème year residents)?

11/ Do you agree that the length of the paediatric residency should be extended from 4 to 5 years?

Yes No Specify why

12/ How many compulsory semesters in paediatric services are you proposing?

6 semesters 7 **semesters8** semesters

13/ How many semesters of neonatology services are required? semesters

14/ Would you agree to a placement in a specialist paediatric department?

Yes   No

If so, for how long1 semester semesters

15/ Which of the following specialised services would you find useful?

Paediatric intensive careYes No 1 semester 2 semesters

Paediatric haematologyYes No 1 semester 2 semesters

Paediatric nephrology Yes No 1 semester 2 semesters Paediatric

gastroenterology Yes No 1 semester 2 semestersPaediatric pneumo-allergology

Yes No 1 semester 2 semesters Paediatric endocrinology Yes No 1 semester 2 semesters

Paediatric OncologyYes No 1 semester 2 semesters

Paediatric NeurologyYes No 1 semester 2 semesters

Paediatric rheumatologyYes No 1 semester 2 semesters

Paediatric emergenciesYes No 1 semester 2 semesters

Metabolic diseasesYes No 1 semester 2 semesters

Paediatric CardiologyYes No 1 semester 2 semesters

Child psychiatryYes No 1 semester 2 semesters

Paediatric SurgeryYes No 1 semester 2 semesters

Other (please specify)

16/ Would you like to do a hospital placement abroad?

 Yes

 No

Why or why not?

17/ Would you like to continue working in a university hospital?

Yes No

If so, which sub-specialty would you like to pursue?

Specify

If not, where would you go from here?

Specify

18/ Overall, how would you rate the theoretical training in paediatrics?

Please select ONE ONLY

 Very good

 Fine

 Insufficient

 Very inadequate Specify why

19/ Overall, how would you rate practical training in paediatrics?

Please select ONE answer ONLY

Very good

Fine

Insufficient

Very inadequate Specify why

20/ What are the shortcomings of your current training?

Semiological collection?

If yes, specify for which complaints? If yes, specify for which contexts?

Clinical reasoning for diagnosis If yes, specify for which complaints?

If yes, please specify for which contexts?

Formulation of a summary of a medical observation If yes, specify for which complaints?

If yes, please specify for which contexts?

Prescription drugs? If yes, specify for which complaints? If yes, please specify in which contexts?

Announcement of a diagnosis to parents and child: If yes, please specify which one(s)?

Education of children and the family If yes, specify for which complaints? If yes, specify for which contexts?

Indication of specialist advice If yes, specify why

Reviewing a medical article

Writing a publication

Technical skills If so, which ones?

Time pressure If yes, explain

Other (please specify)

Evaluation of the paediatric curriculum by teachers

1/ What is your title?

Professor

Associate Professor

Assistant

2/ Gender

Men

Woman

3/ How long have you been with the Faculty?

Over 30 years

25-29 years old

20-24 years old

15-19 years

10-14 years

5-9 years

Less than 4 years old

4/ Are you a framer?

Yes No

If yes

4.1.Are you the only person responsible for looking after the resident?

Yes No

4.2.How did you become a mentor (choice or compulsory training)?

Choice

Imposed

Training

4.3.How many residents do you supervise every six months?

4.4.What is the average number of hours per week reserved for supervisory staff?

4.5.What are the most difficult aspects of your job as a framer? Please explain.

4.6.Do you have any documents or audiovisual material in the company that could make it easier to supervise the trainee?

4.7.Are you relieved of some of your duties to supervise the resident?

4.8.Personally, what do you gain from being a framer?

5/ What learning methods do you use in an internship context?

Presentations

Clinical cases

Indirect supervision

Bibliographic staff

Role-playing game

Other (please specify)

6/ What is your opinion of the current assessment system: a single exam at the end of the course?

	Not at all	Little	Medium	Many	Entirely
Level of agreement					

Suggest improvements

7/ What suggestions would you make to improve the supervision of trainees? 8/ What is your opinion of the current assessment system: a single examination at the end of the course?

	Not at all	Little	Medium	Many	Entirely
Level of agreement					

Suggest improvements

9/ What is your opinion on extending the duration of the paediatric residency from 4 to 5 years?

	Not at all	Entirely
Level of agreement		

Specify why

10/ How many compulsory semesters in paediatric services are you proposing?

6 semesters D 7semesters D 8 semestersD

11/ How many compulsory semesters do you propose for neonatology departments?

1 semester D 2 semestersD

12/Would you agree to a placement in a specialist paediatric department?

Yes D No D

If so, for how long? 1 semester D   2 semesters D

13/ Which of the following specialised services would you find useful?

Paediatric intensive care	Yes No	1 semester 2 semesters
Paediatric haematology	Yes No	1 semester 2 semesters
Paediatric nephrology	Yes No	1 semester 2 semesters
Paediatric gastroenterology	Yes No	1 semester 2 semesters
Paediatric pneumo-allergology	Yes No	1 semester 2 semesters
Paediatric endocrinology	Yes No	1 semester 2 semesters
Paediatric Oncology	Yes No	1 semester 2 semesters
Paediatric neurology	Yes No	1 semester 2 semesters
Paediatric rheumatology	Yes No	1 semester 2 semesters
Paediatric emergencies	Yes No	1 semester 2 semesters
Metabolic diseases	Yes No	1 semester 2 semesters
Paediatric Cardiology	Yes No	1 semester 2 semesters
Child psychiatry	Yes No	1 semester 2 semesters
Paediatric Surgery	Yes No	1 semester 2 semesters
Other (please specify) Adult medicine department Yes D No		

14/ What are your views on training courses for residents abroad?

Yes

No

Why or why not?

15/ Overall, how would you rate theoretical training in paediatrics?

Please select ONLY one answer

Very good

Fine

Insufficient

Very inadequate Specify why

16/ Overall, how would you rate practical training in paediatrics?

Please select ONLY one answer

Very good

Fine

Insufficient

Very inadequate Specify why

17/ What are the strengths and weaknesses of your training as a supervisor?

SUMMARY

Objectives

Involve paediatric teachers and residents in an experiment to evaluate their theoretical and practical training and seek to bring out criticisms, positive or negative, of the current curriculum in order to improve certain aspects of this reform of the third cycle of medical studies in paediatrics.

Study population and methods

We carried out a cross-sectional, descriptive study in the form of a survey of residents and university hospital paediatric teachers.

We included paediatric residents in their 1ère 2ème 3ème and 4ème year, who had completed their medical studies at the 4 Tunisian faculties of medicine, and university hospital paediatricians from the 4 faculties of medicine.

Results

During the study period, we received 50 responses from residents and 40 responses from teachers, representing a participation rate of 29.76% and 50% respectively.

%. Women predominated, with a sex ratio of 0.38 for residents and 0.33 for teachers. Thirty-two teachers (80%) used audiovisual aids in their training. Nearly 90% of the residents said they had received lectures, 68% had taken part in clinical case discussion sessions and 66% had taken part in other learning modalities, eight percent of whom had reported mannequin simulation as a training modality. The majority of participants agreed with the current end-of-specialty evaluation method. However, 26% of the residents questioned opted for formative and summative assessments, and 40% of the teachers proposed an assessment in the middle and at the end of the course. The results of the questionnaire evaluating knowledge acquisition show that daily practice is considered very important for the majority of residents. Theoretical teaching is typically based on clinical cases and lectures. Theoretical teaching in

paediatrics appeared to be insufficiently adapted for 34% of residents and well adapted for 64%. For the majority of participants in our study, practical training is of great importance. It was considered adequate by 72% of residents and 88% of teachers, and inadequate by 28% of residents and 7.5% of teachers. The reasons for residents' dissatisfaction with their training were mainly lack of supervision (33.33%), lack of autonomy and time constraints (9.52%). More than half the teachers were convinced that there was a lack of resources for practice.

Conclusion

Overall, residents and teachers tend to agree with the current learning and assessment modalities of the paediatric curriculum. However, our study has shown that the rapid development of digital technologies has created a need to integrate innovative teaching techniques with sustained clinical activity in the field. This opens up prospects for pedagogical action to improve the quality of training for paediatric residents.

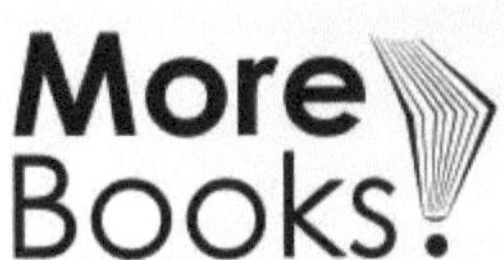

More
Books!

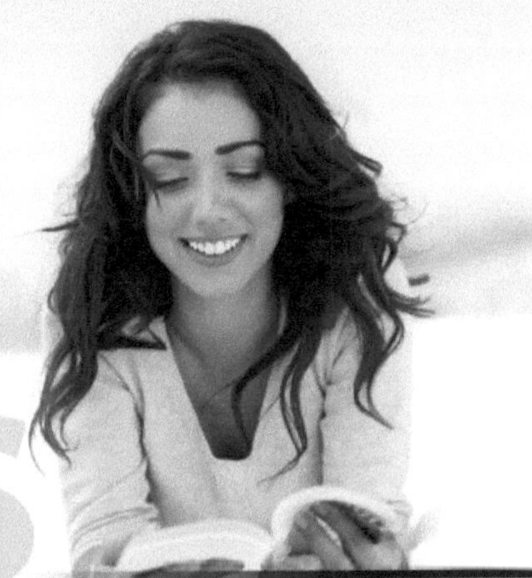

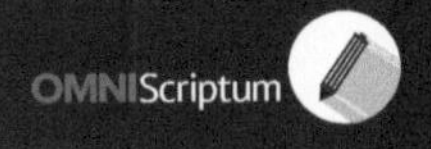

info@omniscriptum.com
www.omniscriptum.com
OMNIScriptum

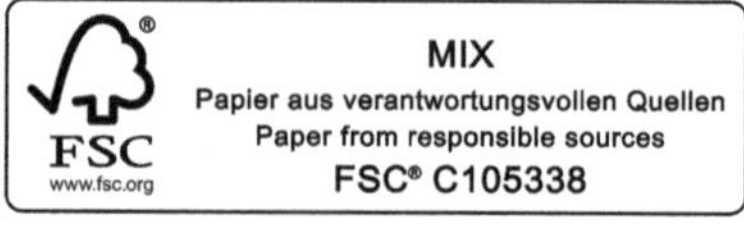

Printed by Books on Demand GmbH, Norderstedt / Germany